I0487346

Living with Schizophrenia

Travis Breeding

ISBN: 1541056159
ISBN-13: 978-1541056152

DEDICATION

This book is dedicated to people who live with Autism. People who live with it each and every day. People that are trying to figure out the unwritten social rules of everyday life. It is also dedicated to the many people who love them. Many people spend countless hours, days, weeks, months, and years working to help someone with Autism. To those of you professionals and parents who are helping someone with Autism m along on their journey. This book is a thank you for everything you do.

The Reality of Living within Two Worlds is also dedicated to my best friend Heather. Heather is one of those people who loves someone with Autism. She helped me along my journey. She stood by my side through some very tough times ensuring that I was strong and able to succeed. This book wouldn't be possible without Heather's caring support and friendship. Thank you Heather for all you have done for me.

CONTENTS

i

Travis Breeding

Autism, Asperger Syndrome, and
Schizophrenia

1 DUAL DIAGNOSIS

Having both autism and schizophrenia

makes many things very challenging for me.

I used to be able to complete and do many

tasks that anyone could do but those simple

tasks have just gotten harder for me to

complete over the past few years. I feel like

the psychosis and the psychotic episodes

are really playing with my brain and they

are causing me a great deal of stress. When

I did not even know, I had schizophrenia I

had always known that I had autism since I

was 22 years old. Having autism is not the

end of the world and it is not nearly as

challenging for me to live with as

Schizophrenia is.

I think that I would do okay in life and be

successful if it was just the autism that I had

to worry about but having schizophrenia

gives a whole new dimension to try and

deal with. Hallucinations and having many

things happen to you that other people do

not see or understand is a very scary thing

and many people do not realize just how

severe my hallucinations and delusions are.

The scariest hallucinations and delusions

are the ones that want me to harm myself.

I try hard to ignore those voices,

hallucinations, and delusions but

sometimes they get the best of me. 25 is a

voice that I hear and he is very mean to me.

He says that I must self-harm because I do

not have a girlfriend and that is very

frustrating because I have tried very

extremely hard to get a girlfriend but having

autism and schizophrenia has seemed to

complicate the issue of dating for me.

Whenever I am alone I hear these voices.

They are telling me to cut my wrists open

and sometimes they want me to remove my

own body parts. There are a lot of voices

that tell me to harm myself but there are

many times when I can fight against the

voices and control them.

I am taking several medications right now. I

take 150 mg of Zoloft, I take 10 mg of Bus

prone, and I take 30mg of Zyprexa. Those

medications sometimes seem to be able to

stabilize my delusions and hallucinations

but sometimes they do not always work as

good as they should.

Right now, as I write this I am hearing

voices telling me that I am not a good

person. The voices want me to punish

myself because I have autism and they are

constantly trying to get me to believe that I

am less than other people because I have

autism and will never be neurotypical. I do

not like hearing voices so I am very relieved

when my medication is working good and

taking care of eliminating the voices for me.

It is very important for me to stay on my

medicine and take it each day. It is

important because if I go a day without

taking my medicine then I could relapse and

have problems with hallucinations or

delusions.

The Ratticle is another name for one of my

voices. Raticle is a boy who makes fun of

me and teases me when I am alone and not

with any other kids. He is always telling me

that I am a dork because I have autism and

he is always telling me that I should punish

myself because I have autism.

Before I started hallucinating or delusions I could cope and live with my autism well. It was not until I started having severe hallucinations and delusions where I started not being able to cope with autism because the voices were making it harder for me to function. By making fun of me and bullying me because I had autism.

Autism is not hard to live with. Surely the Asperger Syndrome in me makes things more difficult but there are a lot of resources to help people with autism. I

have found a lot more autism resources

than I have found resources for mental

illness and I am hoping the mental illness

community rises much like the autism

community did in the mid 2000's. Once the

Autism boom began and numbers of

diagnosed children with autism were to 1 in

150 the autism community started booming

with services and service providers. This is

something the mental health community is

lagging far behind in.

While autism comes easy to me and dealing

with it is easy there are certain things that are very difficult for me when it comes to schizophrenia. Schizophrenia is not nearly as easy as having autism spectrum disorder by itself. Voices and hallucinations are a part of my life but they are not a part of my friends or family member's lives. Therefore, it is hard for me to find someone to talk to that understands how I am feeling or exactly what is bothering me the most. I find that often I must hold my symptoms in and hide them. I try very hard to hide my symptoms because I am afraid of what other people will think if they find out that I

have Schizophrenia.

Both autism and schizophrenia cause a lot

of behavior issues because when you

cannot get your most basic human needs

met in life then there will naturally be some

behavior problems. Behavior problems

with autism can come from just trying to

get your basic needs met in social situations

in friendship and relationships. Not

understanding how to socialize can make it

more difficult for someone trying to live

with autism and it will cause them to

become depressed and feel isolated. Those feelings of desperation can cause someone with autism to start having behavior problems and this is not a good thing.

While someone with autism's behavior issues might be caused by the overwhelming amount of pain and frustration that they face from dealing with real life rejection in the real world someone with Schizophrenia's behaviors are being caused by things that are not even real and do not exist to others in the real world.

Imagine walking the face of the earth each day feeling like someone was wanting to hurt you or target you. Imagine feeling like you were on someone's list of people that they were out to get and find or punish.

Imagine feeling like someone is always watching you or following you. How would that change your behaviors? These are all things that most people only think about but I obsess over because I am constantly having those fears and feelings but I am told by other people that my thoughts and feelings are not real. It is very depressing and frustrating for me to try and sit and

listen to someone tell me that what I am

describing to them is not real. It becomes

so painful that I must punish myself

because I am not able to communicate my

frustrations to other people.

When it comes to punishing myself, there

are only a couple forms of punishment that

the voices want me to do. Many times,

they want me to cut my wrists with a razor

and other times they want me to burn it

with a lighter. They want me to cut and

burn my wrists and I am not sure why. They

say it is because I must be punished for having autism but I do not really want to be punished and I wish that the voices would just go away and leave me alone.

Another form of punishment that the voices try and use is to tell me that I must be punished by removing a part of my body. The worse experience that I have had with Schizophrenia is when the voices will try to get me to remove parts of my body. This does not happen often and has only occurred on two occasions of my life so far but sometimes it is very overwhelming.

In 2012 the voices had me convinced that I had cancer. I was seeing this doctor named Dr. Stankaski and he was trying to tell me how to treat myself for cancer. It all seemed so real to me and he kept telling me that I needed to perform an operation on myself. He told me that I had to remove my thyroid because the cancer was in my thyroid and he was going to guide me on how to do it step by step. I went to what I thought was a hospital and I had real conversations with Dr. Stankaski. I really did believe that I had cancer and he told me how to remove my thyroid. He said I had

to remove about 10 ounces of blood from

my thyroid area to get all the cancer out

and I tried to do this with my razor that I

shave with.

I remember being very scared and nervous

about performing an operation on myself

but Dr. Stankaski assured me that he was

there to supervise and would take over if

anything were to go wrong. Dr. Stankaski.

Later I would learn that none of this was

real and it was only real to me. Others did

not understand why I had tried to remove

my own thyroid and no one understood

that Dr. Stankaski was real to me. He told

me how to do thyroid surgery and I did it

without even thinking about it because it

was all real to me. I went to what I thought

was a hospital but later learned I was

performing the operation at a park on a

bench that I thought was my hospital bed.

The park was not really the hospital like I

thought it was and I remember thinking I

spent several nights in the hospital when I

later learned I was staying the night outside

in a local park sleeping on a park bench.

Schizophrenia can be very dangerous. The whole Dr. Stankaski incident and the thing with trying to remove my own thyroid was my first major psychotic break I think. I was not taking medication for Schizophrenia like I am now and I had no way of knowing that I had even had schizophrenia up until that point when the doctors decided I had psychotic symptoms associated with Schizophrenia.

I always encourage people with

Schizophrenia to take their medications and follow through on their treatment plans. I feel much happier when I am stable and not having periods of psychosis from the schizophrenia. Like I said before I am very capable of living with and coping with the symptoms of autism but it is the psychotic symptoms that come along with having Schizophrenia that gives me the most difficulty.

Autism is not a mental illness and people can work with someone on the autism spectrum to help them learn the necessary social skills that are needed to be able to

function in life. But one thing that you can't

treat without medication is psychosis.

Psychosis is when the brain is not wired

right and there is a chemical imbalance in

the brain. Medicine is a great intervention

for someone suffering from psychosis and it

will help them a lot once you find the right

medications.

I will say for me it has been a mystery and a

real experience in just trying to find the

right medications that work for me. Please

be sure to consult your doctor. You might

even ask them to do a cheek swab that will tell them exactly which classifications of medicines will be of the most benefit to you. It is very important to find the right group of medicines and weigh the side effects of each medication and compare that to the cons of taking that medication.

I feel I am better able to function when I am on the right medications. Sometimes it is hard for me to function on medicine but for the most part I do okay. The only severe side effects that I tend to get from the medications is that it makes me very sleepy and I sleep a lot. I have gone from sleeping

6 hours per night to sleeping for about 14

hours per day. That is a huge increase but if

it is going to help keep me from

hallucinating and delusions then I am all for

it.

Thanks for reading my short story about life

with autism and schizophrenia.

2 PUNISHED FOR WORKING

I was so excited about getting and starting a new job. Autism is very hard for me and sometimes that makes it challenging for me to work and keep a job. As I get older it becomes even harder and I hear voices. I recently was offered a new job and I am so sad because I do not think I am going to be able to take it and be successful at it. I am

already hearing the voices telling me that I

am not good enough for other people and I

am not allowed to work with real people

because I am not a real person because I

have autism.

The voices are very loud and sometimes

cause me a great deal of stress and anxiety.

I take medication for the voices but that

rarely helps me because they are so loud

and overwhelming it is just like they are

trying to hurt me. I do not let them hurt me

and I try very hard not to listen to them. I

like to ignore them because they always tell me bad things. But it is hard for me to be able to focus or concentrate on going to work or having a job when I am just hearing these same voices all day long.

It would be better if I could find a job where I can work in an environment where I am by myself because then there would not be other people around for the voices to tell me that others are better than I am. It would be much easier for me to concentrate and focus on things if I were working in a job where I was by myself and did not have to interact socially with other people.

I was just offered a new job at a factory and I really do want to take this job. But I am supposed to start on Monday and I am already hearing voices about it telling me that I am not good enough to have a job and other people are better than me. I am hearing the voices that are yelling and screaming at me trying to get me to not work. I want to fight them and I am trying to fight them but it is just all too much for me to handle and I do not know if I am going to be able to go to work on Monday.

I really want to work but work has been so

hard for me. I just want to be normal. I

want to have a real job and make money for

myself but that is so hard for me because of

autism and schizophrenia. I hate hearing

voices that try to bring me down and you

would think I would be use to them by now

but it never gets any easier. It only gets

harder. The voices are loud and they are

yelling and screaming at me tonight already

and it is only Saturday. I am very frustrated

and tired of trying to fight the voices but I

know deep down that I cannot give up. I

must be a fighter and I must take on all the

voices. I cannot let the voices beat me and I

will not allow them to define me.

I am going to try this new job because I

know I need the money and I really want

the job. I have never been able to be

independent because of my autism and that

has caused me a great deal of pain. I just

want to be normal and I want people I work

with to like me and I want to be accepted

for who I am. It is so hard for me because

the autism and the schizophrenia have

taken over my life. I am so fixated and obsessed with where I am at in life and I just want to overcome some of my social challenges. I want to overcome autism and I want to overcome schizophrenia. It is just very difficult for me to overcome but I promise everyone I will keep trying hard at this thing called life.

The voices are already telling me that I should punish myself for getting a job. That does not even make any sense at all and I am just unsure of where they even come up with this stuff. They are just so loud and the things they tell me seem so crazy. Why

do they always tell me such crazy things? I

do not understand what the voices want

from me but I wish they could go away

forever and leave me alone. It would be

superb if they could just quiet themselves

and go away and I know that is what the

medication is supposed to make them do

but it just isn't working and it hasn't worked

for over 3 years since I started taking

medications.

I try to learn how to deal with it and just

accept it. It is hard though because the

things they tell me are so loud and

repetitive. I want to fight the voices and I

will fight the voices. I want to be a real

person and have a real job. I want to have a

real paycheck and be a real person. I really

do and I do not want to be called lazy

because I am unable to go to work or keep

a job but it is just all so hard and

overwhelming for me. The voices are

driving me nuts right now and I just want to

go to sleep so that the voices will go away

and leave me alone. The only time I do not

hear voices is when I am sleeping. I have

started sleeping a ton and it is hard for me to wake up in the mornings. I think that is a side effect of my medication honestly and I know I need the medication but sometimes I wish there were not so many side effects to that medication.

Zyprexa is the medication that causes me to sleep a lot and feel lazy. I am not naturally a lazy person but the medicine just makes me very tired and that is frustrating for me. I want to be better and I know I must take the medication to be better so I will just have to deal with the side effects of the medication so that I can live and be happy.

I hate when the voices start talking to me when I am working and I talk back to them. I hate talking back to them in front of other people but it is so hard for me to ignore them. My coworkers or other people around me just think that I am some crazy person but that is not true. It is not my fault that I hear voices or see things that other people do not see. I cannot control it. Sometimes I must talk back to them because of what they are saying. What they are saying is so crazy, loud, and overbearing that it drives me insane to the point that I must stand up for myself and fight back.

I really want to take this new job at a factory that I was just offered and I hope to be able to do so. I know it is hard for me with the voices but I feel like they will go away in time if I can just stick with it and show them up.

If I could just earn a modest paycheck and become independent, it would help a ton. I just need to be given a chance to be able to work. I need to be given a chance in life. I just want to be normal. Somedays I wake up and wish that having Schizophrenia was just a dream. I want to be better and I also want to be neurotypical.

Sure, having autism is not the end of the world. Unless you hear voices that tell you that you must hurt yourself and be punished because you have autism. I am not sure what the relationship is to autism and punishment from the voices I just know that they do not want me to have it. I work very hard at trying to overcome my autism.

I work on social skills constantly and feel like I have come a long way with my autism but the voices just do not want me to have autism. My voices think people with autism should be punished. I have punished myself before because they tell me to.

I am in a fight now because I really want to take that job. The voices tell me if I take that job that they are going to do everything in their power to hurt or punish me. I do not want to be hurt or punished anymore but I really want to take this job and become independent. I will stand up to the voices and I will fight them and beat them. The voices will not hurt me or beat me anymore. I will not let them win the fight.

3 SEXUAL HALLUCINATIONS

I feel like I cannot be a real person because I am a woman trapped in a man's body. I feel like emotionally I am more like a woman than I am a man and this is scary to me but I feel like I am trapped trying to be someone I am not. I am supposed to be a man and be strong but sometimes I have episodes in which I become very emotional and act more like a woman. I feel like I must be a woman because I cannot be a real person by being a man. I am not able to feel a woman's breasts because I do not understand social and emotional connection. I feel like I cannot be accepted for who I and I believe that because I am trapped inside the body of a man when really, I am a woman.

It is hard for me to focus because I can't stop obsessing over this thinking that I am not a man and am instead a woman. I feel like if I become a woman I will not have to be a bother to anyone else because I will be

able to experience many of the things that I

need to experience because I will already be

a woman and I will be able to experience

what being a woman is like. I will have my

own body that would be like a woman's

body and it would not be hard for me to

connect with myself like it is for me to

connect with other women.

Having autism and schizophrenia just

confuse me greatly and I want nothing

more than for it to go away but it is not

going away and it only continues to get

worse. I just want all the pain to stop but it does not stop and it keeps getting worse. Each day goes by, the pain gets deeper and deeper and no matter how much I try I am not able to experience a woman and that really hurts me and makes me want to become a woman.

I am stuck here and in a trap and I cannot get out. Will someone let me out please? I cannot live with myself because I am not a real person because I am a man and not a woman. It is very important for me to be able to become a woman because I cannot be a normal person as a man.

I have a disability as a man and I hope that by being a woman I would not have a disability any longer. I have felt confused about my sexuality for a long time and I have been confused as to why other women do not understand me. I am not sure why other women do not understand me and it makes it hard for me to be able to fit in because no one wants to accept me for who I am. Most men do not accept me nor understand me at all. Most women do not understand me at all. I have one good friend who is a woman that gets me and cares about me and that helps me cope with things to the best that I can.

I fight the voices every day. Most days' voices tell me that I need to have a sex change and become a woman. I hate hearing these voices. I think deep down I really want to be a man and I really want to be able to be accepted as a man. I really want to be understood and I want others to like me and I wish that this could happen as a man but I do not think it is possible for me to be liked and accepted as a man. I feel I must have a sex change and become a

woman so that I can be accepted and loved.

I do not think that I can be accepted as a

man. I feel like the only way to happiness is

to become a woman and to have a sex

change.

I feel that having a sex change will help me

with a few things. First it will help me to be

able to experience sex and sexuality on my

own without having to rely on other people

or women to help me have sexual

experiences. It will be easier for me to

experience having female body parts and

expressing myself and enjoying them

because I will not have to go to someone

else and get them to like me or accept me

to connect with them on that level to be

able to experience things.

If I can just become a woman my life will be

real and I can be a real person but there is

no way for me to become a woman because

I do not have the money to be able to do

that and my insurance will not pay for any

procedures to help me become a woman.

My insurance won't even pay for a dating or

relationships coach to help me understand

woman so I am very frustrated and feel as if

I am stuck or trapped here on this earth.

There is something severely wrong with me

because I have Schizophrenia and I

constantly hear and see things that other

people do not experience seeing or hearing

and it makes me feel like I am a weird

person but I just cannot help but to wonder

what my life might be like if I was a woman.

Would I be less weird or awkward if I was a

woman? I am not sure what to think but I

know it is very painful for me to be a man

and I would hope that it would be less

painful for me to be a woman than it has been for me to be a man.

I feel like I am not a real person. Why do I always feel like a fake person? I must be real but I do not feel like things about me are real. I feel like I am living in a different world than the rest of the population is and I fear that people are out to get me. I must hide myself and stay in my house to be safe. I must be able to turn into a woman so that I can protect myself from the bad people that are out to get me. I just must be able to get away. I must run and hide I just cannot stay here as a man anymore which is why I would hope that I would be able to have a sex change and become a woman. I think I would be safer here on earth as a woman than I am as a man and I think women would understand me better as a woman and maybe even other men would relate to me better if I was a woman.

I often hear voices that tell me I must do bad things to myself. Luckily, I can tell that these are just stupid voices when I am on my medication. I can fight off the voices when I am on my medication and that really helps me cope. I take so much medicine that I feel like I am a medicine cabinet. I feel like if I don't take my medicine that I will die.

I just have never been accepted as a man. People say you must love yourself before other people can love you but how is that even possible? I do not understand how I can love myself when other people do not love me. I feel like I need some sort of evidence that I can have as proof that I can love myself. I need approval from other people so that I can be liked. I just need to be loved and accepted but it seems like that is impossible.

Sometimes I get random letters that come in the mail that people swear they did not write. Sometimes I hear voices saying these bad things. Sometimes I hear voices telling me that I must punish myself because I am a man and that is why I want to become a woman so that I can make the voices happy. The voices yell and scream at me reminding me that I should be punished because I am a man. I do not understand why the voices are so mean to me and yell at me in this manner but I hope one day to be able to be accepted and at this point and time I feel like the only chance that I will ever have to be accepted is if I become a woman and get a sex change.

It is so much easier for me to talk to women and relate to them than it is for me to talk to other men and relate to them. Men are too worried about being tough and cool and care too much about their image. At least women like to talk about things that I enjoy talking about and can relate to them about. Women are very complicated and I know that if I were to become a woman I would

probably be the most complicated women

in the world but at least I would not have to

be punished anymore for being a man. I

hate when the voices tell me that I must

punish myself for other people to like me.

It is my hope that if I become a woman that

I will not have to punish myself anymore.

The voices tell me I must be punished

because I cannot see or feel breasts. If I can

become a woman I will have my own

breasts and I will not need to be punished

because I can see and feel my own breasts.

I think we all want what we cannot have and that is very challenging for me. I have been wanting to be loved and accepted for a long time but it is so hard for me because I am a man and I have autism. It is hard for me to focus because these thoughts have become very intrusive and they make it so I am unable to think clearly. The voices and hallucinations are present nearly every day of the year and sometimes they get tiring and I just want a break.

My medicine does help but it makes it hard because the medicine makes me very tired and lazy and sometimes all I want to do is

sleep. Sleeping is peaceful because I am not

hearing all the voices, seeing ghosts or

spirits, and I am not seeing or hearing

anything. Sleeping is peaceful and I enjoy it

very much but I fear that I am missing out

on life by sleeping so much. I wish there

was a way for me to be awake and not hear

voices or see things that others do not see

but it just might be my reality that I am

always going to hear voices and see things.

However, I do think that becoming a

woman would solve a lot of my issues and

cure me from autism. I feel like becoming a woman would make my autism invisible. I feel like people would not notice that I was as different if I was a woman and I feel like someone would be able to love and accept me for who I am if I were a woman.

I know that becoming a woman will not solve all my issues but I do feel like it would help me to be loved and accepted. I hope one day I am either cured from autism or become a woman so it is easier for me to be loved and accepted.

4 SEX WITH A MENTAL ILLNESS

Having sex is a very intimate thing between

two people but when a third person is

present it makes having sex more difficult.

This is the case for me having

schizophrenia. It is very hard for me to be

able to focus on anything throughout my

day because I feel like my brain is just that of a video game playing. I am constantly hearing things and seeing things that other people do not even begin to comprehend. It is so hard for me to function and even difficult for me to get and keep a job. I have not experienced a lot of successes in my life due to the voices, hallucinations, and delusions that are pretty much ruining my life but I try hard to overcome them.

Having autism and schizophrenia it is very difficult to function in social relationships until you get to the point where you can have sex with someone. You must really

develop a relationship socially and try to get

to know someone before you have sex with

them and it can be hard to get to know

someone when you just keep hearing voices

that tell you that you are not good enough

for other people. It can become very

frustrating and lonely. I remember the first

time that I was in a sexual relationship. I

could not even sit with the girl I was with

without hearing voices. The voices would

tell me that I was not going to be good

enough and they said I was a failure and

would not allow me to be successful.

The first time I went to kiss a girl I immediately started hearing voices trying to tell me I was doing it wrong. Wherever I go and whenever I am with other people I am never alone. There is always another person around me or beside me trying to get me to believe that I am not a good person. It could be Milky the cat trying to tell me that I am not a good person and it can be Dr. Stankaski and it could also be Tom who is trying to tell me I am not a good person.

Whenever I am cuddling with a woman I

have random women that I like that just

show up and try to prevent me from

cuddling or having an appropriate time with

the woman I am with. I hate when voices

show up in the form of women I have liked.

It is hard for me to function when I keep

hearing the women tell me I am not good

enough for the woman I am with and the

voices will also tell me that I should be

punished for trying to be with the woman I

am with. The voices always want me to

punish myself because I have autism. I am

not sure why but the voices do not like

autism and they are always trying to get me

to hurt myself.

I want them to leave me but it is like I am

infected with voices. The voices are mean

to me and I do not often hallucinate that

are nice to me. They just keep telling me

repeatedly that I must hurt myself because I

am autistic. They tell me that people with

autism are not allowed to have intimate

and sexual experiences. The voices say I

must cut my wrists with a razor anytime I

engage in an act of intimacy with someone.

I wish the voices would leave me alone because I am a real person and want to be a real person. The voices keep reminding me that I am not a real person because I am autistic and that really hurts my feelings. I just want to be like everyone else and all people would like to have romantic experiences or intimate experiences. It is important that we help people with autism develop social skills necessary to navigate social relationships that will lead to intimacy and sexual experiences for them.

When I try to cuddle with a woman they

keep telling me that I am not doing it right

and I am not going to do a good job. I get

very nervous and anxious when I am around

other people because the voices make me

fear that I am messing up or making

mistakes. I try not to listen to them and

sometimes people will reassure me that I

am doing okay but those voices and

hallucinations are so overbearing. I just

wish that they could stop and not be so

annoying at times.

I want to focus. I just want my brain back. I

want to be able to concentrate on what I

am doing but it has become so hard for me

to do that because of the voices and

hallucinations. I do not know what else I

can do or try. I try to ignore them but the

voices are in my head all day and night and I

just want to be left alone. Especially when

it comes to being with a woman. I would

like to be able to enjoy an intimate

experience and cuddle with someone

without having to worry about voices,

hallucinations, or delusions trying to

interfere with my experience. It is already

hard enough for me to be intimate with

someone because of the autism that I have.

I just wish the voices did not exist because

they always tell me that I am not good

enough for other people.

There are a lot of girls I like. Sometimes I

get letters in the mail from girls I like asking

me to punish myself because I am autistic. I

do not understand why these girls want me

to punish myself but I ignore them and try

not to harm myself. It is very important

that I ignore what the girls are telling me.

These letters are from real women that I

like but they do not necessarily know that I

like them so I know that someone is telling

them that I like them and that is the reason

why I keep getting letters from them. It is

very scary to get these letters asking me to

cut myself or harm myself. I refuse to give

into them and I refuse to listen to them as

they do not always know what they are

talking about.

It is so hard for me to enjoy my life and any

intimate experiences that must do with life

because I am unable to focus on anything

because the voices refuse to leave me

alone.

I want to make sure my girlfriend has the best time of her life so it is important for me to ignore the voices. The voices are very loud and disturbing and cause me to feel depressed and anxious. I just want to be able to have a few days in my life in which I do not hear voices. It has become an every-day thing and I take a lot of medication to help with it but still sometimes it is hard.

Imagine trying to have sex with a third person or a ghost standing over you talking to you and telling you that you are doing something wrong every step of the way.

That is what a sexual and intimate

experience is like for me.

5 NEGATIVE SYMPTOMS

I had to do it. I had to hang myself. The voices were yelling at me and screaming telling me that I needed to try to hang myself. Whenever I hear those loud voices I get really scared and am not sure what to do so I need to rely on my friends and family to help me cope with these voices of destruction.

No one knows why I hear voices or see

things that other people do not and there is

not much we can do about it to help me

other than making sure I am taking the right

medication every day of the week. It is very

important that I am taking the medication

as prescribed by the doctor so that I can be

sure that I am treating the psychosis and

voices.

Why are there never any nice voices? Why

are all the voices so negative and

destructive? Why do they want me to harm

myself? I will never understand but it is like

my brain is this constant video game of messages going back and forth. It is hard for me to know if what is happening in my brain is real or not so I am often asking people if what I am experiencing is really happening just so I can be sure.

This past week I have heard voices telling me that I must hang myself because I have autism. For some reason, all my voices are about trying to get me to punish myself because I have autism. The voices are so loud and overwhelming and they just want me to harm myself as a punishment for being autistic. It is very challenging because the voices will even tell me that other people I want to be friends with or date want me to harm myself because I have autism. It is very scary and real to me but no one else can understand what I am experiencing. I am sad that no one else understands what I am going through and I just wish that other people would be able to learn what it is like to hear the voices that I hear.

I think the voices are getting worse the older I get because they tell me more bad things now than they ever have before.

Now they are always trying to get me to

hurt myself and they want me to do bad

things to myself. I am glad they do not ask

me to do bad things to other people

because I could never live with myself if I

hurt someone. I need to be able to stay on

my medication to help make sure that I am

always able to function.

It has become increasingly difficult for me

to be able to work because the voices want

me to hurt myself and I often hear voices

telling me that the people I work with are

trying to hurt me. Like right now I am

conflicted because I really want to get a job

and I do not know if I am going to be strong

enough to be able to fight off the voices. I

have tried many jobs and have never had a

problem with physically doing a job but I

really struggle with being able to navigate

social relationships on the job probably

because of my autism and schizophrenia

both. It makes sense that it would be

difficult for me to function in social

relationships because of having autism but I

think the greater difficulty for me comes in

the way that the voices and hallucinations effect my social relationships.

It is also scary when voices try to convince me that there are chips inside of me and want me to try and cut the chips out of my body. Like right now the voices are telling me there is a chip in my brain and I should try to open my head or skull with a knife and cut the chip out of me. Luckily because I am on my medicine I can tell that that is just a voice in my head and not something real that I am experiencing. It is very hard and overwhelming to live with this but I am trying to stay positive and make the most out of a bad situation.

While the medicine helps, me realize that the voices are not real and that I am hearing things in my head I do not feel as if the medicine is doing anything to stop the voices or to keep them from talking to me. I hope one day I find the right medication to either make the voices stop or at least get them to say good things about me instead of saying bad horrible things about me.

Sometimes I hear voices from the television

and my family tries to convince me that what I am hearing the people on television tell me is not something that is real or something that everyone hears. They tell me to do bad things to myself. Sometimes the news anchors on the nightly news tell me to do bad things to myself like cut my wrists or burn myself and I have a hard time coping with that. It is very hard for me to be able to understand what I am going through sometimes. Sometimes I do not know what is wrong with me and when I am experiencing psychosis it feels like I am an alien or some fake person trying to live here on planet earth but then other times when I am not experiencing psychosis it feels like I am always depressed because I am very aware of my situation. It breaks my heart to think I might have to live with this for the rest of my life but then I want to make sure I am doing everything in my power to be happy and live a productive and amazing life. I really need to work on trying to be more positive during the downtimes when I am not having psychosis so that I can start to enjoy life again.

I am still adjusting to my new diagnosis and it will take some time but I hope one day I will be able to say that autism and schizophrenia are not running my life. There is no disorder or disease that will run my life because I will take ownership of these disorders and make sure that they do not interfere with my life. Thanks for reading my frustrations tonight.

I tried to hang myself because I thought other people wanted me to hang myself based on the voices I was hearing. I wish I did not have bad voices telling me that everyone is saying bad things about me but

I do and I am trying to learn to cope with

that. I am very grateful and fortunate that

someone could find me and prevent me

from killing myself. I was very lucky and

have a very caring family and friendship

circle.

6 SERIOUS HALLUCINATIONS

Today I am feeling very overwhelmed. I have autism and schizophrenia and I have a lot of intrusive thoughts going through my mind. The voices really bother me and hurt me. I just wish the voices I hear in my head could stop or go away. I do not know why they continue to yell at me and bother me.

They are so loud.

Sometimes I am confused on if the voices are really voices or if they are just deep intrusive thoughts that I am hearing in my brain. I just know that they are super loud and sometimes it feels s like they are screaming.

Today the voices are telling me that I need to self-harm. Luckily, I am doing better and am taking medication so I am not listening to them. The voices say that I need to try and cut autism out of me with a razor blade. The voices do not like the fact that I am autistic and they always want me to try and cut so that I remove the autism and I receive my punishment for having autism. It is very difficult some days to argue with the voices because they are very loud.

I do not know how to make the voices stop. Taking my medication seems to help a little bit but they are always there. I have not had many days in which I have not heard voices for a very long time. It is like they live with me and are a part of my life but no one else can see them. Why are the voices so loud and more importantly why do they always want me to do something to hurt myself?

One of my scariest hallucinations is when I hear voices that try to tell me I should light myself on fire. This one voices I have named Tom thinks that I need to light myself on fire and be punished because I have autism. Tom always tries to give me instructions or directions on how to light myself on fire. He wants me to get inside of my truck and use a gas can to light a match and burn myself alive. That is a very scary hallucination I have but I try to ignore him and the medicine is helping me do that some.

Why does Tom want me to hurt myself? I have never done anything to him but he always thinks I need to cut or self-harm or even blow myself up with a gas can in my car. Tom is mean and I do not care for him. I wish there would be nice voices sometimes too that did not tell me to cut myself or hurt myself. I always ask my doctor why the voices cannot be nicer and say good things instead of saying bad things.

Schizophrenia is very hard to overcome and people who love people with schizophrenia must be very patient with us. It is hard when you constantly have voices because it is like there is a video game playing in my head. Thank you for reading this short story about what living with schizophrenia and autism is like.

7 POSITIVE SYMPTOMS

I am so paranoid about everything. It always feels like everyone is out to get me and conspiring against me to try and hurt me. When I try to go to work I hear voices telling me that I am not good enough to be working with the other people that I am working with because I have autism.

It is extremely challenging for me to go anywhere or even just to leave my house because I am constantly having this thought of paranoia where other people are going to be waiting on me outside of my house to try and hurt me as soon as they get the chance.

I am always hearing voices that tell me that people from the state and the autism non-profit organizations in the state are trying to harm me and conspiring against me because I have high functioning autism and I have a mental illness.

As soon as the autism non-profits in my

state found out that I had a mental illness

they stopped talking to me and told me that

they could no longer help me and that

really hurt my feelings. I cannot help it that

I got sick and have schizophrenia or a

mental illness but it seems like the autism

non-profit organizations are constantly out

to hut me. I feel like the leader of the

autism non-profit organization in the state

of Indiana is trying to make other people

hate me because I am high functioning.

The autism non-profits always seem to

favor people who are lower functioning and

have more severe problems than people

like me who are high functioning.

I just always thought that the autism non-

profits would be able to help all people with

autism. When I have made suggestions to

try and get the autism non-profit

organizations to advocate for different

services that I think I need and would help

me to become more successful socially and

ease my depression and anxiety they have

come back and told me that the services I

am asking for are not medically necessary.

I am not sure how anyone other than the patient would be able to say what is and is not medically necessary but it really hurts my feelings that the autism non-profit organizations do not see the importance in social intervention

I am so scared to leave my house that I cannot even work or go to school. Any attempt to work or go to school has always been unsuccessful for me. Mainly, because I am constantly hearing voices that tell me I should not be leaving my house because as soon as I leave my house someone will be waiting outside to hurt me in some way or form. It is very hard for me to function in life and the mental illness or the schizophrenia seems to have taken over a lot of my life and is really making it hard for me to be successful in anything I do.

I am so paranoid about someone trying to hurt me that sometimes it is hard to even eat my meal or enjoy my dinner. I try hard to not let this paranoia affect me but it is so hard. It is even hard for me to take my medication for schizophrenia because I am constantly hearing voices that tell me that the autism non-profits and the state are trying to poison me.

The only way I can take my medication is because I know deep down that the medication can make these voices say better things or sometimes it can make it so the voices do not say anything at all and that is amazing when that happens.

Many people do not understand paranoid schizophrenia. The fear is real and it is active. My own family for example has a hard time understanding why I am unable to go to work and unable to function

normally. They do not understand the

amount of stress that I am under since I

hear voices and see things that others do

not. I live in a constant state of fear and

that is scary.

Sometimes I like to just sleep so I am not so

paranoid and I take some medications that

help me so that I am better able to relax

and fall asleep. Before I took sleeping

medications, it was always very difficult for

me to fall asleep because I was afraid that

someone would try and hurt me if I was

sleeping.

It does not matter what I do or where I do it I have these constant voices and am scared. I tried going to new places at one point in my life thinking that it would make things better and I would be able to function better in life but the voices and paranoia only followed me everywhere I went and made it worse.

There was a time when I used to enjoy my life. I remember a time when I did not have this paranoia feeling and was not afraid of anyone or anything. I remember a time when my brain was free of voices saying terrible things about me and I remember a time when I could go to school and work without fear of being hurt.

It is emotionally exhausting for me to have these feelings all day long because it is like my brain never rests. I want my brain to rests sometimes so I do not have to be anxious and living in a constant state of fear of being hurt. It is so hard for me sometimes because I struggle with social skills and social relationships anyways because of autism and the symptoms I suffer from schizophrenia just make that struggle worse.

I want the voices to stop so I take my medicine but they do not always stop. Sometimes I am scared to go to the doctor because I am afraid that the autism non-profit organizations will try and hurt me. It is very scary knowing that my doctor can prescribe me medicine to help me but sometimes it is hard to go and see him because I am afraid he will try and poison me.

Schizophrenia seems to have taken over my life and these hallucinations and delusions have really begun to interfere with my ability to enjoy life. I just wish that there was a cure for it so that I did not have to suffer from the voices and hallucinations and delusions.

I am constantly afraid and paranoid of everything. Even the slightest noise can really bother me now. I used to like loud music but now I cannot stand it One day I hope to be able to play trombone again and join a band but right now I just could not handle it.

If you have not lived with schizophrenia you are lucky. It is hard and it is important to have a friend network and a supportive family that supports you.

I do not know if my paranoia will ever go away but I hope one day I can lead a normal life, maintain a job, and be a functioning member of society.

ABOUT THE AUTHOR

I enjoy camping, hiking, backpacking, and traveling. I hope to visit all 50 states one day along with traveling abroad. I like meeting new people so I go to new restaurants and hot spots throughout the city from time to time. I also have numerous online friends in which I stay in touch with through social networking sites

like Facaebook and Twitter.

I am a sports fan. Football and Basketball

are my favorites. I play some recreational

sports for fun only. I root for the IU

Hoosiers, Boston Celtics, Green Bay Packers

and Indianapolis Colts.

I have Asperger's which just means I'm

Awesome. My friend told me to write that.

If you have questions about it, just ask me.

Having Asperger's also means that I'm nice,

smart, super trustworthy, love to tell the

truth, but I can sometimes seem a bit

forward.

BIBLIOGRAPHY

Living in a Make-Believe World

Travis shares what living in his make-believe

world is like as it helps him cope with social

situations and autism. He uses the make-

believe world sparingly as a tool to help him

be happy and successful socially and

emotionally. Learn how his make-believe

world works for him and against him as he

thrives on living with autism like a trooper

in this great book about a young man living

with autism.

Travis tells all in this amazing read that is

sure to put the reader inside the mind of

someone with autism and allow them to

experience autism like they are in an autism

stimulator. If you have ever wondered what

it is like to live with autism then you must

read this thrilling and suspenseful book

about what it is really like to live in a make-

believe world that others do not

understand and succeed with autism.

Travis was always different growing up but

today he sees his autism as a blessing and

something to be thankful for. Now Travis

hopes to help others understand him and

the interesting traits of autism so that the

world can be a better place for all people

affected by autism and improve the quality

of relationships between the autistic and

neurotypical person. Read this book to live

and experience autism like Travis does.

"This is one of the most moving accounts of

growing up with Undiagnosed AS that I have

read. Travis Breeding's honesty and

willingness to share his struggles with some

of the obstacles he faced growing up is a

treasure trove for anyone on or off the

spectrum. If you have a friend or family

member who is different from what you or

society expects, this story offers a bird's-eye

view of what it might feel like to be in their

skin." Maripat Jordan Robison

Becoming a Social Thinker

"Context is King" is a quote by Dr. Peter

Gerhardt a Behavior Analyst in the field of

Autism. Understanding context is critical for

social success. Communication is 93 percent

non-verbal and it is important to use our

social thinking skills to be able to read and

understand social context and social

dynamics. Learn how I taught myself to

become a good social thinker by studying

good body language.

This book will teach you everything you

need to know to become a good social

thinker. You will learn how to read and

decode body language and facial

expressions to get a full picture of what

people are trying to communicate with you.

You will also gain the ability to read and

understand social context or social

dynamics in social settings.

In a world where communication is 93

percent non-verbal and only 7 percent

verbal it is important that we get a full

picture of what people are trying to

communicate to us. This book will help you

learn how to read what other people are

trying to say and help you communicate

who you are in a more advanced way that

will allow others to see you for who you

really are.

This is a great book for parents and professionals wanting to gain better understanding into advanced social concepts like social thinking and the ability to read and decode body language and facial expressions. This is also a great book for adults and teens on the autism spectrum to read in order to become better at understanding social thinking and social context.

How to Love Your Autism

Travis shares how he learned to love his autism and himself during this amazing story of how a man received several medical diagnosis as he struggled to accept and love himself. He shares that learning to love himself might have been the greatest disability that he faced. Loving ourselves takes time and patience and that is something Travis does not have. Will he fall in love with himself again?

In this story you will find out if Travis is able to fall in love with himself again like he did as a child. He will take you through the ups and downs of Autism, Schizophrenia, and Hydrocephalus to show you how he overcame blaming Autism for all of his problems. It is helpful to have a complete full picture of your medical issues when judging what is causing you to experience what symptom. Travis shares how a lot of what he thought was Autism acting up was really Schizophrenia and Hydrocephalus working together to make him miserable.

Travis uses Cognitive Behavior Therapy with the help of his new counselor to form more positive thoughts about himself and his autism. Letting go of something is a hard thing for someone with a mental illness to do. Travis takes you through his battle with his greatest enemy which is himself in this amazing book on what life with Autism, Schizophrenia, and Hydrocephalus is like for him. This is a highly educational read that is sure to help teachers, professionals, and

parents understand Autism, Schizophrenia,

and Hydrocephalus a little better.

Autism at the Casino

Travis shares how he made frequent visits

to the casino to help him cope with autism.

Travis thought he could get rich and pay

everyone to like him and not worry about

being socially awkward. His frequent trips

to the casino only caused him more

problems and landed him in a heap of
trouble. He developed an addiction and a
whole host of other problems from visiting
the casino that he copes with.

Travis spent many years thinking getting
rich would solve his problem of making
friends and allow people to love him for
who he was. Little did he know that all he
needed to do was love himself and embrace
who he was in order to get others to love
him. Travis spent years looking for solutions

to his problems on the outside when the

answer was right in front of him. All he

needed to do was improve his self-esteem

and learn to like himself for who he was.

Follow along as Travis turns to outside

solutions like going to the casino to solve

his social issues related to autism. Will

Travis finally get the help he needs from

counseling and learn to love himself or will

the casino get the best of him and cause

him to go bankrupt and end up ruining his

life? This is an action packed true story of

how a man with autism became confused

and started looking for solutions to his

autism in all of the wrong places.

25 Days to Live

True story about how Travis' voices tell him

he has 25 days to live and must lite himself

on fire on December 31st, 2016 as

punishment for not having a romantic

experience with a woman. Travis shares his

voices and hallucinations to help the reader

understand how serious of a mental illness

schizophrenia is. Travis will rely on his

friends and family to help keep him alive on

December 31st, 2016.

Travis talks about figuring out his life after

receiving four major mental health

diagnosis and autism. Travis is learning how

to embrace his challenges and fall in love

with autism all over again. Travis shares

how his friends and family help him fight

the voices and beat them on a daily basis.

Voices that tell Travis to self-harm because

he is autistic must be rebuked and defeated

constantly.

Travis shares how the voices are counting

town the days until he is supposed to

punish himself for not having romantic

experiences with women in this book. He

also shares how he plans to fight the voices

and stay alive past December 31st, 2016.

Travis shares his goals and ambitions for life

after December 31st. He plans to defeat

the voices, continue taking his medication

and get as much help as he needs to live life

to its fullest.

Read this book to see what it might feel like

to have constant voices, hallucinations, and

delusions telling you to punish yourself and

kill yourself. Travis shares how he copes

with schizophrenia and provides many

useful tips for dealing with and fighting

mental illness. He also provides tips and

valuable insight into living with autism that many parents and professionals will find useful. Read along to see how Travis plans to spend what the voices say are his last 25 days fighting the hallucinations and improving his quality of life.

The Apology

Travis writes a heartfelt apology to the autism community for the way he behaved in the past due to his mental illness that magnified autism issues and made autism

appear to be worse than what it really was.

Now that Travis has answers and a full

picture of what he is dealing with he is

ready to apologize and correct the mistakes

he made in the past and make things right

with everyone he wronged.

Travis shares how autism is not an excuse

but a reason. Travis was diagnosed with

Schizophrenia in 2013. That diagnoses

would give him many answers as to why he

had been behaving the way he was. It is hard to control your behaviors when you are hearing voices, having hallucinations, and experiencing delusions. Travis was convinced that he had to pay women an autism bill in order to like them and get them to like him. He became so desperate to pay what he thought was his autism bill that he began stealing money from his parents, extended family, and friends.

Travis was in a fight for his life to stay alive.

Fighting suicidal ideation for years Travis

tried to get rich so he was able to pay his

autism bill and did not have to kill himself.

Travis opened a publishing business to try

and help parents of children with autism

share their stories with the world but ended

up mishandling business money and having

to file for bankruptcy with his business.

Travis ended up not being able to provide

the services people paid him for because he

used the money to pay people to hang out

with him.

Travis is in the process of making things right with everyone who was wronged through his business and he is in the process of paying back his family and friends for all of the money he took from them. Now that Travis has a full and complete picture of his mental health he knows that Schizophrenia is not an excuse for poor behavior but a possible reason for his irrational thinking and behaviors.

Travis feels relieved to learn that the

majority of his problems are not likely

autism related but more so related to

schizophrenia. With a comorbid diagnoses

Travis hopes to apologize to everyone that

he hurt by being selfish and stealing money

to pay people to hang out with him. If you

or someone you know gave Travis money

and feel that you did not receive the

services you paid for Travis will encourage

you to reach out to him in this book so he

can make things right with you. Read the

book for instructions on how to contact

Travis so that he can make things right with

you.

This is an honest and caring book written by a guy who really cares about other people and wants to make a difference in the world. The best thing you can do is learn from your mistakes and Travis feels like he has learned from his mistakes. He is now ready to move forward with his life and help others understand autism and mental illness by sharing his stories and knowledge with the world.

How to Improve Your Autism Services

Travis shares tips and strategies to help improve your child's autism services to ensure they get what they need out of their treatment plan. He stresses the importance of treating social thinking like an adaptive living skill so your child will can communicate with others both verbally and non-verbally as an adult. This book will be useful in helping you advocate for your child.

Travis shares his experiences with self-advocacy and talks about how you can train your child's staff to help them best meet your child's needs. Travis shares that communication is seven percent verbal and ninety-three percent non-verbal. Most services are designed to work on verbal or adaptive living skills but ignore non-verbal or social thinking skills. Travis teaches the reader about social thinking and how it comes into play in all social aspects of life.

Using the Facebook green dot as an example Travis will break down a social skill and show you the verbal and non-verbal components of each skill. Verbal means adaptive and non-verbal means social thinking. Travis will provide valuable insight as an adult with Asperger Syndrome into how the mental health system and service providers can best help your child with autism providing the insurance industry allows them to do so. This book examines

how to save America money in the long run

by providing early intervention and non-

verbal social skills training to people with

autism spectrum disorder. This read is sure

to help parents learn to be the best

advocate they can be for their child on the

autism spectrum.

Autism or Autistic

Travis addresses the issue of if he is an

autistic person or a person with autism.

Travis says it is not important to him what

you refer to him as if you get to k=now him

for the person he is instead of the

diagnosis. He does not let labels bother or

define him. So many with autism make a big

deal out of the name of the label that they

fail to realize they are a human being and

not a label.

Travis worries that people with autism have

been misled to believe that their diagnosis

is their core identity. While Travis strongly

believes, autism is a part of who he is, he

does not allow it to define him or put

limitations on his life. Travis wants to

improve his social skills to have a better

quality of life, not to change who he is.

Travis feels improving his social skills will

help him better communicate who he is to

others and allow him to feel more

understood for the person that he is.

Travis talks about how he will not allow the

words you use to describe him affect him as

he continues to learn social skills to be able

to better communicate with others and

improve his quality of life. Travis talks about

why it is hard for him to make friends with

other adults on the autism spectrum and

provides insight into how Asperger

Syndrome comes into play with his

personality. Travis feels it is important for

counselors to stress that autism is s part of

who someone is but should never be their

core identity. Travis says if a person

believes autism is their core identity it will

be hard to ever help that person because they will worry that you are trying to change who they are.

Travis examines the obsession with wording of a person with autism versus an autistic person in this informative book that will give insight into the way someone on the autism spectrum views himself. Travis says the most important thing is that there is a human being on the inside of the label on the container. Travis hopes to learn social skills that allow him to show others who the

human being is on the inside of his

container.

How to Drive a Car with Autism

Travis provides powerful and moving insight

on how to teach someone with autism to

drive a car safely. Travis gives several teach

for teaching the adaptive living skill of

driving a car responsibly while teaching the

reader how to teach someone with autism

the social thinking skills to navigate traffic safely. Never has there been a book that can help you teach someone with autism to drive.

Travis covers everything in this book from teaching someone with autism how to steer, shift gears, accelerate, and brake. He will also give tips and ideas to help someone with autism learn the rules of the road. Travis says driving is a lot like socializing. Driving the car is the social skill and communicating with other vehicles are the social thinking skills and non-verbal communication skills. Using turn signals is a form of non-verbal communication as are break lights. To be a good driver you must learn how to read all the written rules like stop signs and traffic lights and then improve your driving skills by learning how to read the unwritten rules or the non-verbal communication from other drivers.

Travis provides tips for preparing your son

or daughter for interacting with the police if they get pulled over and provides a step by step guide for how to teach someone with autism what to do if they encounter a traffic accident without having a meltdown. This book will be extremely helpful for parents who are worried that their child with autism may never be able to drive and live independently. Travis shares his story of how he learned to drive to provide hope and inspiration for people with autism and those that love them.

How to Like Someone with Autism

In this book, Travis explains how his brain works like an on and off switch. He shares how that causes him to either be all in a friendship or not in at all. The problem is when he goes all in it is too soon and it scares people away. This is particularly common in dating relationships as Travis has struggled with coming on too strong and scaring women away. This makes Travis feel bad and confused.

Travis shares how he works very hard on social skills and learning unwritten social boundaries and rules so that he does not scare women and other people away. Travis becomes very fixated on people and sometimes the person turns into a special interest. We are familiar with children with autism having a special interest like that of Thomas the Train or something like that. What we are not familiar with is when adults form a special interest in another person that they can obsess over.

Obsessions and fixations can create many problems for someone on the autism spectrum. It takes intense behavior therapy to lessen the obsession or fixation. Travis works hard with his therapist to control the fixation or obsession with other people. In this book, Travis, will teach you how he is learning to cope with and overcome the fixation and obsession with getting to know other people. Travis gives tips on how to help improve social relationships for someone on the autism spectrum so that they are more likely to be accepted and

liked by their peers.

This is a great book for parents and

educators looking to get directly inside the

mind of someone living with autism. Travis

explains his thought processes on

friendships and relationships. This book will

be a useful resource in helping you work

with people on the autism spectrum.

How to Make Friends with Autism

Learn how someone with Autism makes friends and analyzes friendships through social thinking. Travis shares his experiences in building meaningful friendships in this great book about friendship with autism. Learn how to use social skills to meet people and form friendships in socially acceptable ways that draw people to you instead of pushing them away. You will learn to make and keep friends in this inspiring tell all book about how a man with Asperger Syndrome or Autism makes and keeps his friends.

Travis writes about many of the challenges involved in keeping friendships for him as he overcomes autism related issues and social thinking errors. Friendship is all about communication and studies suggest communication is ninety-three percent non-verbal and only seven percent verbal. In this book, you will learn how Travis works with social skills coaches to learn the ninety-three percent of non-verbal communication so that he will be able to better

communicate with his friends and have an

everlasting meaningful friendship with

them.

Travis talks about the many issues that

might come up in a friendship. You will

learn about sensory issues that can make a

person on the autism spectrum

uncomfortable in social situations and

friendships. You will also learn some useful

strategies in helping to motivate someone

with Asperger Syndrome or Autism to want

to make friends. This is a great first-hand

account about what it is like to make and

keep friends for someone on the autism

spectrum. This is excellent reading for

parents of children diagnosed with Autism

and professionals who work with those on

the autism spectrum.

Autism Conspiracy Theory

Travis blows the whistle on the insurance

industry's plot to cover up effective

treatments that help people with autism.

Travis explores why insurance companies

are doing everything in their power to not

pay for applied behavior analysis and social

skills coaching for children and adults on

the autism spectrum. Travis shares how

corporate greed has gotten in the way of

helping people with autism in this

enlightening book.

Travis has fought his insurance company for

years to get them to cover social skills

coaching and applied behavior analysis so

that he can learn the basic social and life

skills he needs to be happy and successful in

life. Travis shares how he has been made

fun of and bullied by his insurance company

for wanting to experience trying social skills

coaching to learn social skills to live with

autism to the fullest. Travis talks about the

hidden conspiracy theory and the greed of

the insurance industry that is keeping your

loved ones with autism from getting the

help they truly need.

In this book, Travis, will provide the reader

with useful information and tips to fight

your insurance company for better autism

related services and treatments. Travis

exploits the hidden conspiracy of corporate

greed by leading insurance companies in

the United States of America. Included in

this book is a bonus section on how to live

with autism during the holiday season.

Travis provides tips on helping your loved

one with autism enjoy the holiday season

and everything it must offer in this very

informative book. This is great reading for

parents and professionals who work with

people on the autism spectrum and deal

with insurance companies.

www.ingramcontent.com/pod-product-compliance
Lightning Source LLC
Chambersburg PA
CBHW071433180526
45170CB00001B/333